Communication

A Reflective Guide To Mastering Communication Abilities
And Enhancing Social Abilities

*(Technologies Are Revolutionizing Corporate
Communications)*

Desmond Sutherland

TABLE OF CONTENT

Introduction

A couple who had been together for several years existed once upon a time. They were deeply in love and spent the majority of their time together.

One day, the couple decided to discuss sexuality. They had never really discussed their sexual desires or expectations, and they were both apprehensive about taking the plunge.

The male initiated the conversation by inquiring about his partner's desires in the bedroom. She responded that she desired to feel desirable and appreciated. She also desired to feel that her companion was attentive to her needs and desires.

The fellow was taken aback by her response but was willing to engage in conversation. He shared his own thoughts and desires with her, expressing his desire for her to feel

1

protected and valued. He also wanted her to share her fantasies with him so that the experience would be pleasurable for both of them.

The couple communicated with complete candor and without any sense of humiliation. They discussed their preferences and fantasies and were able to find common ground.

The couple felt more connected and in harmony with each other after the conversation. They were able to investigate their sexuality because they had created a safe space for communication.

Sexual communication is the exchange of information, thoughts, and emotions regarding sex, sexual health, and sexuality. It includes talking about sexual activity, contraception, reproduction, sexual orientation, gender identity, and sexually transmitted infections (STIs). It consists of both verbal and nonverbal communication, such as body language, contact, and facial expressions.

Sexual communication is crucial for a healthy sexual relationship. It can increase intimacy and mutual understanding between partners and reduce the likelihood of miscommunication or misunderstanding. It can also help to develop trust and consent by ensuring that both parties are clear on their desires and consent.

Physical autonomy is an essential component of erotic communication. This means that both partners have the right to consent to or refuse any sexual activity with which they are apprehensive, regardless of the opinion of the other partner. It is essential to remember that consent must be freely and without coercion given. It is also essential to communicate honestly and candidly with your partner about any feelings of discomfort or uncertainty.

Additionally, it is essential to comprehend the significance of boundaries. This implies that partners should respect one another's right to privacy and personal space. This includes respecting each other's right to decline participation in any activity that causes discomfort.

Other essential components of sexual communication include discussing contraception, STI prevention and testing, and emotional security. In addition to discussing pleasure and gratification, it is essential that both partners feel heard and respected.

Overall, successful sexual relationships require effective sexual communication. It serves to increase understanding and trust, and can reduce the likelihood of miscommunications and misunderstandings.

It is essential to remember that individuals have varying comfort levels and requirements. Respect your partner's sentiments and boundaries by being open and honest about your own. Partners can create a safe and enjoyable sexual experience through open and truthful communication.

Managing Difficult Individuals

When working in a team, you will encounter a variety of personalities, some easygoing and others not so much. Personality issues that are not addressed can have disastrous effects on a team, leading to increased tension and conflict.

After identifying the type of conflict using one of the methods described in the preceding chapters, there are a variety of approaches to address the tension. Analyzing how various personalities manage conflict will also provide insight into how to approach it.

Utilize preventative measures; when you recognize that tension is escalating within your team, address it before it becomes a significant issue, at which point it will be more difficult to resolve. When you observe that one of your members is irritated, communicate with them to give them the opportunity to discuss the issue before it escalates.

Maintain the harmony; continue to listen to your members, as they may feel that their input is not being considered. When you sense your heartbeat increasing, take a deep breath and remind your teammates to do the same. This will also prevent more furious words from being spoken, preserving potentially salvageable relationships.

Give the team a chance to discuss the issue, concentrating on the facts as they explain their respective perspectives.

As described previously, brainstorming is an effective method for your team to generate ideas for resolving their conflict. This will also give them new perspectives on their coworkers and methods to interact with them.

Empathy is essential because it enables you to comprehend the perspective of your teammate. It will provide insight into the conflict's true nature and why your team member reacted as they did. It will also enable you to identify and discuss growth-promoting solutions.

Finding a method to work through a difficult situation with personalities who find it difficult to express themselves positively can reduce tension and minimize flare-ups in the team, creating a more enjoyable work environment.

Chapter 1: How to Effectively Form Your Message to Get Your Point Across

Have you ever been uncertain about how to initiate a conversation? If you have, you have likely missed out on excellent potential conversations. Imagine you want to speak with someone, but they do not make eye contact and appear uninterested in conversing. You may feel unwelcome and believe that it is difficult for them to attend to your story. Or you may be conversing with a person and ponder if you should mention the most recent film or book you've read.

Consider a time when someone did not make eye contact with you or their responses seemed sluggish. How did they respond to your remarks? Was their body language accommodating? If not, what was their response?

Remember their response, and then use this information to maintain your relationship with them in future conversations. Consider, the next time a close friend or family member approaches you to speak, what approach worked best for them in your current situation. Did you make a noteworthy remark? Did you make them laugh? How could you make their next visit more enjoyable or meaningful?

What are some frequent errors that people make when communicating with others? What behaviors do some individuals engage in during conversations that drive away observers or create an awkward situation?

We all experience communication problems at some stage in our lives. Even if we have developed exceptional communication skills, people will not always comprehend us as we intend. Communication is bidirectional, so we must ensure that both parties are understood.

Here are some helpful suggestions on how to effectively structure your message.

1) Seek clarification if you desire a second opportunity to convey your meaning. The first thing that comes to mind when considering requesting clarification is a student who repeatedly poses the same question to their teacher. No matter how frequently you ask, this individual will not remember what you said or how to respond to your inquiries. Even if you ask them multiple times to clarify a basic question such as "When did Ike become president?" they may still not comprehend the situation.

2) Stick to a single topic: When engaging in conversation, lie back, relax, and focus on the other person's responses. Do they respond enthusiastically to your

comments? If so, you are fortunate. If their body language is hostile, defensive, or uninterested, refrain from pressing the issue. The more you demand their attention and insist on your point, the less receptive they will be to your message.

3) Tell them what you want from them: "I want to speak with you about something that can have a significant impact on our lives." This demonstrates that you have at least one topic in mind and requests the audience's input. In addition, it demonstrates to them how important the matter is to you.

4) Listen to the other person: Conversationalists will find a way to make everyone they converse with feel at ease. If you are interested in what they say, pay close heed to what they say. If you are only concerned with communicating your ideas, it will be difficult to determine what they want or how their ideas may influence yours. This can damage a relationship because

friends and family don't like feeling like their personal space is being invaded, and they will pressure you to leave.

5) Learn how to say "no" (without coming across as impolite): Learn how to say "no" as soon as you recognize that the topic may not be interesting or relevant for the situation and audience. The purpose of saying "no" is to let them know that it is not a good time to discuss that topic and to assist them in moving on to something that may work better.

6) Plan your remarks: what can you say that will be meaningful and engaging? You may not even be able to communicate your intended message. Before speaking, it is ideal to have a few prepared lines or ideas. If you are unprepared, it is easy to engage in a rambling conversation that lasts longer than it should.

7) Know when to halt and allow the other person to speak. You may wish to respond to what the other person says, but you must listen first. This often

necessitates a little amount of time to formulate your thoughts and comments. When it comes to initiating your thoughts, don't rush. Give yourself as much time as necessary, especially if the other person is speaking quickly or their words appear to be rushed.

8) Refrain from interrupting. The simple rule is that if someone's comments confuse you or seem out of place, you should give them an opportunity to present their thoughts before interjecting your own. People appreciate it when someone takes the time to consider what they want to say, demonstrates patient, and refrains from interrupting them when they are speaking.

9) Consider the manner in which you express yourself: There are two components to the message you are conveying. The first component is what you say, and the second is your delivery. This can include your body language and voice tone. You should ensure that your

words match your tone of voice and body language. If someone appears angry, ensure that the tone of your message reflects their voice or body language. Ensure that your message suits the facial expressions and overall disposition of a person who appears cheerful.

10) Maintain eye contact: Frequently, individuals will not speak with us if we do not maintain eye contact. They may even request that we look aside if they are uncomfortable with our gaze. When communicating with another individual, there is no need to avoid their gaze by staring at the ground or the center of their face. Maintain appropriate eye contact by concentrating on the individual's eyes.

11) Be honest: If you are dishonest, you cannot anticipate a positive outcome from your conversation. If you lie, it will likely come across in your speaking tone and body language, making the other person feel uneasy around you.

Maintaining positive relationships with others requires honest and open communication.

12) Avoid being judgmental: No one wishes to be evaluated based on their opinions, thoughts, and emotions. If you believe that someone is incorrect or that their perspective is overly idealistic, you should carefully consider your response. The best method to respond could be to simply state, "I see where you're coming from, but I must express my disagreement." You could also say, "I disagree with that thought because of this reason. Try not to judge what they say or paraphrase their beliefs in an offensive manner. If you cannot do this, it is best to keep your thoughts to yourself and not engage in a lengthy defense of why they are incorrect.

13) Utilize the individual's name to demonstrate your interest in them as a person. Additionally, you can use their name in your comments or responses to show that you are paying attention to

what they are saying. You are not required to use the other person's name in every other sentence, but you should include some references that honor their identity.

14) Refrain from performing multiple tasks during a conversation: Be present and attentive to the other individual. You may have things happening in your life, but you must temporarily set them aside in order to have an intimate and meaningful relationship with the individual you are speaking with. If you choose to act as if there is something more essential than conversing with someone, you should not be surprised if they appear upset or offended by your words. They do not overlook these issues because they desire a healthy relationship with someone who cares about them.

Chapter 2: The reasons behind stage anxiety

There are numerous potential causes of stage fright, which is a prevalent form of performance anxiety experienced by many people when delivering a public speech or presentation. Among the most frequent causes of stage anxiety are:

If a person lacks confidence in his or her speaking abilities or subject knowledge, he or she may experience nervousness or anxiety.

Fear of failure or negative evaluation: Individuals may worry about making errors or being negatively evaluated by their audience.

Lack of familiarity with the audience or topic: Speaking to a new or unfamiliar audience or about a topic that is outside of one's comfort zone can cause anxiety.

Symptoms: physical Physical symptoms such as a rapid heartbeat, profuse sweating, and trembling can also contribute to stage anxiety. The release of adrenaline in response to tension or anxiety may be the cause of these symptoms.

Previous unpleasant events: Past negative experiences with public speaking, such as feelings of embarrassment or humiliation, may also contribute to stage anxiety.

Individuals can develop strategies for managing and overcoming stage anxiety if they are aware of its causes. Numerous individuals find it beneficial to familiarize themselves with their material, rehearse their delivery, and employ techniques such as deep breathing or visualization to calm their nerves. Seeking support from friends, colleagues, or a professional therapist can also be useful in managing stage fright.

Typical stage anxiety symptoms

When giving a public speech or presentation, performance anxiety, also known as stage fright, is a common occurrence for many individuals. Among the most frequent indications of stage fright are:

Increased heart rate: Stage anxiety can result in a faster heartbeat, which can be uncomfortable and distracting.

Anxiety can cause an increase in perspiration, resulting in clammy palms and forehead.

Shaking or trembling: Stage anxiety can result in physical tremors, such as shaking hands or a trembling voice.

Anxiety can cause a dry mouth, making it challenging to enunciate or swallow.

Difficulty thinking: Stage anxiety can cause a person to feel overwhelmed and unable to think clearly, making it challenging to recall what to say or do.

As a result of anxiety's somatic effects, some individuals may experience nausea or an upset stomach.

Anxiety can cause shortness of breath, resulting in feelings of distress or discomfort.

These symptoms may or may not be present in every instance of stage fright, depending on their intensity. While stage fright is a normal and prevalent experience, it can be managed and overcome through practice and preparation. Numerous individuals find it beneficial to familiarize themselves with their material, rehearse their delivery, and employ techniques such as deep breathing or visualization to calm their nerves. Seeking support from friends, colleagues, or a professional therapist can also be useful in managing stage fright.

Chapter 3: What is the definition of effective leadership communication?

Certain individuals appear to be born pioneers, while others are forced to take initiative. History demonstrates that many individuals with truly humble beginnings have emerged from nowhere to become legendary figures. What distinguishes Julius Caesar and Napoleon? What makes Richard Branson, Steve Occupations, and Warren Buffett resemblances in the modern era, with less fighting?

One thing they all have in common, practically speaking, is that they are persuasive communicators, or "turn specialists" They comprehend the significance of imparting a dream that people must continue to pursue. Julius Caesar and Napoleon both mastered deceptive publicity and had the ability to convince the public that their defeats were actually victories.

Powerful contemporary pioneers such as Branson and Occupations constructed organizations without any preparation, with every worker convinced of the mission's significance and willing to do their part.

Each opportunity for authority will involve obstacles, traps, and arduous periods in addition to triumphs. It is the manner in which a person responds to these difficult periods, and to the numerous pundits who want to dissect them, that can be indicative of an exceptional leader.

Similarly to numerous aspects of ordinary life, timing is also essential. Figuring out how to effectively communicate with your chosen audience in the most eloquent manner and in the most advantageous settings can be difficult, but it can yield enormous rewards.

Consider Your Audience's Perspective

Understanding your audience's perspective is the most important aspect of effective correspondence. This audience will change, so adaptability in one's correspondence styles is a crucial skill for any leader. In a single day as the leader of a company or division, you could address:

Staff Shareholders

Business associates

potential business associates

Vendors Customers

Children taking a tour of your facility...plus much more.

How you address the recipient and what you choose to say or not say are crucial components of effective correspondence. For example, you would not discuss your Q4 sales results with your children. In addition, you would not distribute departmental surveys to your clients, but rather to your personnel.

Appropriate Timing

Timing is likewise important. For instance, no business leader anticipates delivering bad news, but sometimes the longer you avoid it, the worse things can become. In the event that there is a lull and you need to get cutting off workers, this should be communicated quickly.

The Correct Fashion

Using the example of delivering bad news, you must also choose your second and correspondence style. Would it be prudent not to communicate with anyone other than those receiving the formal notice? Emailing everyone? Or, would it be preferable for you to send an email to set a date for an important gathering?

How might you convey the news to the group if everyone is present? Do you merely announce that there will be budget cuts and stop there? On the other hand, will you make sense of the reasons for the decision, the subsequent steps, and your thought process moving forward?

Listening is just as important an initiative skill as speaking. Will you provide employees with access to information about the layoffs and the situation in general? Or forward it once more to your directors?

After the gathering concludes, you will have a variety of subsequent advancements and options. Will you address each recipient of the formal notice, or will your recruiting director do so? Or, alternatively, will these experts be removed without anyone expressing regret or gratitude for their previous efforts?

Sometimes correspondence, for better or worse, results from not expressing anything by any means. A worker who receives a formal notice but is not given explicit reasons or thanked is likely to feel significantly more dejected than one who is treated as an individual.

Chapter 4: It permits companions to support one another

One of the exciting aspects of having a partner is that you always have someone to rely on when facing challenges.

It would be a detriment to yourself if, when you are experiencing difficulties, you chose not to communicate with anyone, particularly your partner.

You may be missing out on the opportunity to find someone whose shoulder you can lean on.

It can be troublesome if your partner doesn't know that you're experiencing difficulties alone.

You may be relationally stunted and mentally disparate at the moment, which can spark disagreements and preferences.

On the other hand, illuminating your partner assists them in comprehending and concentrating on you.

It is an excellent mood enhancer.

In the event that you cannot express your thoughts openly and honestly in a relationship, you have a problem.

One of the goals of a healthy relationship is for partners to freely share their thoughts, concerns, and emotions with one another, without fear of rejection. Legitimate and effective correspondence enacts this statute.

When you share your happiness with a companion, it improves your disposition because the environment becomes less stressful. A secure relationship is one in which both parties master the complexities of effective correspondence.

Instead of "That was courteous of you!"

Attempt: "When that young man collapsed, I saw you assist him. He must have been extremely irritated, right? However, I believe that by giving him a hug, you helped him to feel significantly better. It feels better to aid individuals, doesn't it?"

Again, this relates to observing what your child has done and communicating to them that you have observed and appreciated their activities by depicting what you have observed. Requesting that the child contemplate how they feel about their positive actions as a whole increases the likelihood that they will be repeated in the future.

Instead of: "Yahoo, you pooped in the toilet!"

Try this: "You defecated in the toilet! I'm aware that you tried a few times today but were unsuccessful, but all of your practice has helped, hasn't it? Now you've discovered how to make it happen!"

Potty training and acclaim will often remain closely linked, but praising children for their 'accomplishments' can backfire in this case. First, they may exert themselves to complete a task when they do not have to. Here, the recognition can assist them in ignoring their body's symptoms and eliminating them in order to be commended. This is not exactly what is required for toilet preparation.

Related: Ten positive nurturing techniques for child restraint

Second, applauding results overlooks all the effort put in, regardless of whether they were unable to complete a task or make it to the bathroom on time. However, it is this effort that brought them to their destination. Indeed, regardless of errors, focus on the work itself and not the outcome.

Instead of "Yahoo, you've finally finished your dinner!"

Try: "I assume you're not anxious right now; that's fine. I'll put this food in the microwave; let me know if you want me to reheat it up for you later.

Perhaps the most counterproductive praise is commending for consuming. It encourages adolescents to stop listening to everything their bodies are saying. They discover that it is beneficial to eat when they are not anxious to please others and to consume foods they could do without in order to feel significantly better. Over time, these eating behaviors can quickly lead to bingeing, comfort eating, and dining at home. Keep praise far away from the dinner table.

Instead of "Great job on quieting down!"

Attempt: "Were you actually frantic? It is acceptable to be angry at times. You will develop more techniques for

31

maintaining composure as you age. Up until then, I'm anxious to help you quiet down."

Complimenting children when they are "great" and ignoring them when they are "terrible" can lead to a variety of problems. When infants are frantic, they do not lose their temper for no apparent reason. They're angry because they're not feeling better, and they have no control over their emotions. Loading up on praise when they are silent is like telling them, "I really like you."

Chapter 5: Considerations for Improving Communication Abilities

Below are the top ten reasons why you and your children should develop strong communication skills.

1. Your marriage

According to the National Center for Health Statistics, ineffective communication is the leading cause of divorce for nearly half of all couples. Moreover, if you only consider the Christian community, this number does not change. Nobody can anticipate always getting along with others. The key to an enduring relationship is not conflict avoidance, but rather effective conflict resolution! Men and women communicate exceedingly differently and often for a variety of reasons. This is covered in the first chapter of my book, "Say What You Mean Every Day," titled

"How to Talk to Your Spouse 'Cuz You Must!"

2. Your Offspring

Parents who communicate effectively with their children raise children with defined boundaries and a sense of security. They venerate them and instill in them a sense of worth and value. Strong communication skills allow children to express their requirements and desires. Those who do not resort to violence to satiate their misinterpreted desires.

Your Ministry 3.

What is the harm in inaccurately describing Jesus to someone? They might always decline, correct? Wrong!

A person who has been repeatedly warned that they will be damned to damnation may tire of being spiritually chastised by others. They form a negative opinion of Jesus, Christianity, and Christians in general as a result. Others who identify as Christians may disagree with your viewpoint.

Your friendships, four.

People who are effective communicators value the following: 1) self-assurance; 2) leadership; 3) personal presence; 4) credibility; 5) the ability to explain and persuade; 6) comprehension of others; and 7) the enjoyment of interpersonal interaction.

All of these characteristics enhance our ability to establish and maintain friendships.

5. Your Contentment

Studies indicate that those who communicate effectively are happier than those who do not. This is due to the fact that they have more satisfying careers, marriages, friendships and connections, higher revenues, and more satisfying personal lives. They are able to effectively communicate their requirements and desires, allowing them to obtain the things they want and require in life.

Due to the prevalence of miscommunication and misunderstanding in today's complex and secular society, greater communication skills are required for survival. In addition, mastering each aspect of communication requires a unique set of skills and techniques.

How to efficiently manage customer service, complaints, and refunds, How to contact individuals, Utilizing social networking sites to effectively juggle work and children. When and how to communicate your business beliefs, How to Request Assistance from Friends and

Family, How to motivate your staff, manage concerns with customer relations and corporate image, and educate customer service employees;

All of these issues necessitate a certain degree of communication expertise!

Chapter 6: Comprehending the Advantages of Negotiation

Negotiation is an essential skill to possess in any circumstance where two parties have opposing viewpoints. Understanding the other party's perspective, working together to find a solution that works for both parties, and compromising when necessary are all elements of negotiation. Learning the advantages of negotiation can assist individuals and organizations in resolving conflicts amicably, communicating effectively, and constructing stronger relationships.

When two parties are able to negotiate, they can consider solutions that are beneficial to both. Negotiation permits compromise and innovative problem-solving, which can result in a win-win situation for all parties. In addition to fostering mutual trust and comprehension, negotiations facilitate future communications.

Additionally, negotiations assist individuals and organizations in resolving conflicts amicably. Parties can avoid costly and time-consuming litigation and preserve their relationships by engaging in dialogue to determine the source of the conflict and then collaborating to find a solution. Importantly, negotiations enable both parties to be heard and respected, which is essential for effectively resolving conflicts.

Effective communication is another crucial advantage of negotiation. By engaging in an open and sincere conversation, parties can ensure that their ideas and perspectives are heard and considered. Parties can clarify their positions, pose questions, and exchange ideas in order to reach a mutually beneficial agreement through negotiation.

In any circumstance, negotiation is a valuable skill to possess. Individuals and organizations can learn to compromise, communicate effectively, and resolve conflicts amicably by grasping the benefits of negotiation. Negotiation is a potent tool for fostering improved relationships, establishing trust, and locating mutually beneficial solutions.

Clarifying objectives, identifying common ground, and establishing ground principles prior to a negotiation.

Several crucial measures must be taken prior to the actual negotiation in order to successfully prepare for it. Clarifying objectives and expectations is essential for ensuring that all parties have a shared understanding of the desired outcome. Identifying common ground and areas of accord can contribute to a more productive negotiation atmosphere. Establishing ground principles for the negotiation process can help ensure that the conversation remains respectful and on-topic. In addition to defining the boundaries of the negotiation, ground rules can provide a framework for keeping the conversation on track. In addition, preparing for negotiation entails researching the other party's interests and requirements and gathering any pertinent information that could be useful during the negotiation process. Taking the time to properly prepare for a negotiation will help to ensure that all parties can reach a mutually beneficial agreement.

Utilizing Techniques to Ensure a Successful Negotiation: Establishing rapport, practicing active listening, and employing open-ended inquiries.

For a negotiation to be fruitful, it is necessary to employ specific strategies. Establishing rapport is one of the most vital techniques. This involves establishing rapport with the other individual and demonstrating interest in their viewpoint. Additionally, it requires being deferential, receptive, and genuine. This fosters an atmosphere of trust and mutual comprehension, which is crucial for a successful negotiation.

Active attentiveness is an additional crucial skill. This indicates that you are paying close attention to what the other person is saying and considering their perspective. This ensures that all parties are heard and their ideas and opinions are considered.

Lastly, using open-ended questions to conduct fruitful negotiations is an effective strategy. Open-ended questions are those that necessitate a response other than yes or no. They permit further discussion and exploration of ideas, which contributes to a more successful and fruitful negotiation.

Utilizing these strategies can make the negotiation process more successful and fruitful. By establishing rapport, actively listening, and asking open-ended questions, you will foster an atmosphere of trust and mutual understanding and ensure that all parties are heard and their ideas and perspectives are considered.

Communicating with family and friends

Here are some different points for communicating with family and friends:

Use open and honest communication: Be open and honest with your family and friends, and share your thoughts and feelings. This can help create a sense of trust and understanding.

Practice active listening: Pay attention to what others are saying and show that you are engaged in the conversation. Avoid interrupting or multitasking.

Use "I" statements: Use "I" statements to express your own thoughts and feelings, rather than blaming or criticizing others. This can help you stay calm and focused on your own perspective.

Show empathy: Try to understand and relate to the feelings and experiences of others. This can help strengthen your relationships and build trust.

Respect boundaries: Respect the boundaries of others and be considerate of their feelings and needs.

Seek support: If you are having a difficult conversation, you may want to seek support from a trusted family member or friend.

Effective communication with family and friends involves being open and honest, practicing active listening, using "I" statements, showing empathy, respecting boundaries, and seeking support when needed. By following these tips, you can improve your communication skills and strengthen your relationships with loved ones.

Chapter 7: How To Communicate With Children Of Various Ages

Effective communication with children is necessary for effective parenting because it fosters relationship development, trust-building, and problem-solving. However, communicating with children of different ages can be challenging due to the fact that their communication needs and abilities vary depending on their developmental stage. Due to the fact that children of varying ages have varying needs, interests, and communication methods, parents must adapt their communication strategies in order to successfully communicate with their children and meet their needs.

The use of age-appropriate language and explanations is one method for parents to effectively communicate with children of varying ages. For instance, it may be advantageous to use simple language and provide concrete examples when communicating with a young child in order to facilitate their comprehension of abstract concepts. As the cognitive capacities of their children increase with age, parents may use more abstract language and discuss more complex concepts.

Parents must actively attend to their children and take an interest in what they have to say. This may aid in the development of trust between parent and child. Parents must be patient and provide their children with the necessary time and space for self-expression.

In addition to adapting their own communication style to meet their children's needs, parents may employ a variety of strategies to facilitate effective communication with their children. For example, parents may express interest and support through nonverbal cues such as body language and facial expressions. They may also encourage their children to express their thoughts and feelings by posing open-ended questions.

Using a real-world issue as an example, here are some suggestions for communicating with children of varying ages.

Infants aged 0–2 months rely heavily on nonverbal cues such as body language and facial expressions to develop their social and physical skills. You can help your infant develop communication skills by paying attention to their signals and engaging in activities that encourage social connection, such as singing, reading, and playing peek-a-boo.

As you endeavor to place your infant down for a nap, they begin to cry. Instead of immediately picking them up, observe their nonverbal cues to determine if they are famished, tired, or in need of a diaper change. After attending to their immediate needs, you should attempt to lull them to sleep with a beloved blanket or toy, a gentle touch, or a soothing voice.

Toddlers (2 to 3 years old). At this age, toddlers may have a limited vocabulary and are still learning how to express their thoughts and feelings through words and actions. As a parent, you can facilitate the language development of your children by conversing with them frequently, using simple language, and reiterating words and phrases to help them acquire new vocabulary.

Your young infant is frustrated because you are unable to provide them with the desired item. instead of stating it immediately, try to understand their perspective and affirm their sentiments by saying, "I can see that you want that item. Although it appears to be enjoyable, you cannot interact with it. What if we find you another object to play with?"

Preschoolers (ages 3-5): Preschoolers become more independent, improve their social skills, and may have a greater understanding of cause and effect at this age. You can improve your children's communication and problem-solving skills by encouraging them to express their thoughts and feelings and assisting them in resolving disagreements.

Imagine that one of your preschooler's items has been stolen by a friend. Instead of intervening, encourage your child to speak to their playmate and come up with a solution. You could say, "You appear to be upset because your friend swiped your toy. Can you discuss your emotions with your friend and seek a compromise so that you can share the toy?"

Children of school age (6 to 12 years): At this age, children can engage in more complex conversations and are developing their critical reasoning skills. By asking your children open-ended questions, encouraging them to express their opinions, and listening to what they have to say, you may aid in the development of their communication skills.

Your school-aged child is upset because he or she was not invited to a classmate's birthday party, as in the following scenario. Try to comprehend their perspective and validate their feelings by saying, "I see your perspective" or "I understand why you're upset that you weren't invited to your friend's party." It may be difficult to feel excluded. What, in your opinion, can we do to assist you feel better about the situation?"

The parent may engage the adolescent in a more in-depth discussion about the significance of handwashing and personal sanitation. The parent may also discuss the significance of handwashing in preventing the spread of disease and its potential neighborhood effects.

Successful communication requires being aware of the needs and abilities of children of all ages, actively listening, and providing guidance and support as their communication skills develop.

By implementing these suggestions, you can nurture enduring, uplifting relationships with your children and provide them with support as they navigate the challenges of growing up.

Tools / Formats for Effective CC Strategy

Video Formats and Tools

Video formats such as Vlogs, etc. are rapidly supplanting conventional internal communication tools such as the internal newsletter. It has improved recall and attention capacity, particularly for millennial workers.

Post-pandemic, video conferencing is the new standard for conducting business with both employees and customers. It enhances collaborative communication, reduces time and travel expenses, and boosts productivity.

Every organization should invest in time- and cost-saving tools and platforms.

A growing number of organizations are utilizing video for induction, training, process/policy updates, and safety regulations.

Senior Management can access and record video formats for HRM or change management initiatives even when they are physically unavailable due to travel or other circumstances.

It is also an excellent resource for Project Management Teams that require comprehensive and consistent information.

Videos can be delivered on demand and in real time to meet the requirements of employees. These can be saved to Intranet or Vlogs for subsequent viewing to fill in any gaps, if any.

We can measure audience engagement through analytics monitoring, which is the best feature.

City Halls:

Town chambers promote an inclusive culture and community development. It is by far the most effective and influential format for fostering company culture.

It facilitates direct communication between leadership and employees and aligns employees with the organization's objectives.

In addition, it promotes a culture of appreciating successful employees and learning from errors.

Virtual Events: Virtual Events platforms are cost-effective and facilitate the scheduling of events in a brief period of time for a larger / global audience with minimal resources.

Webinars have a greater audience reach and facilitate audience engagement. Additionally, digital tools enable efficient lead and data collection.

Chapter 8: Entertaining And Exciting

The audience's ability to perceive my passion for the industry when I speak on radio or television is, in my opinion, one of the reasons for my success. This is impossible to deceive, and attempting to do so will result in certain failure. Consequently, your chances of success will increase if you sincerely enjoy your work and communicate this enthusiasm to the people you interact with. I have observed this across a broad spectrum of professions. like former presidents Bill Clinton and Tommy Lasorda.

I spoke with President Clinton during the commemoration of his first year in office at the White House, and he expressed the same sentiments regarding national leadership. Both Clinton and Lasorda are outstanding orators. I've always appreciated conversing with these individuals. Because they all share the same trait—

enthusiasm—in both their work and social interactions. When they interact with a person, they are eager to express their excitement. This has led to their complete achievement in business and in their respective careers.

You probably do not want to encounter failure like Tommy Lasorda. I pray that will not befall any of us. However, life is not always joyful. Not always are we privileged. When something goes wrong, attempt to forget about it and concentrate on the positive. Your family and friends idolize you, as do your interests and charity work. Even something as simple as recently witnessing an engaging film or reading a good book... Rekindle your enthusiasm and joy so that you can always converse with a smile on your face.

If you come across a topic that interests you, try to engage the individual who is listening. This demonstrates your accomplishment.

The Three Exterior Obstacles

Just now, we examined four internal obstacles to communication. Obviously, this list is not exhaustive, but it does provide insight into how our communication is hindered by internal factors.

Now we will discuss the three external barriers. These are the environmental factors that influence our interpersonal communication. External obstacles are problems that occur beyond our control. We may perceive them as occurring "to us" and feel powerless to alter the situation.

1. Social influence

Social influence refers to the manner in which our thoughts and actions are modified to conform to the expectations of a social group, perceived authority, or social role. In other terms, we seek acceptance. Regarding communication, this is a thought-provoking concept to consider. The majority of us recognize social influence. Daily, we are exposed to it via email, social media, mobile phones, etc. But few have considered how it manifests in personal relationships.

For instance, your closest friend calls and asks you to attend a party with them. Due to your familiarity with this friend's partying habits, you are aware that there will be excessive drinking, wild sex, and narcotics at this party. Your friend is aware that you do not drink, engage in public sex, or use illegal substances, but they still invited you. They also mentioned a number of additional attendees. They desire that you serve as the designated driver. You typically serve in this capacity, but recently you've noticed that the gatherings have become increasingly unruly, and your friend's behavior at these events has become increasingly erratic. You do not mind being the designated driver, but it is becoming tedious. Due to the fact that multiple friends are attending, they are each calling you separately to invite you to the party. This is how social influence manifests itself in our daily existence. It is so common and can appear inconspicuous, but it can have a significant impact on our interactions with one another. Because it is easier, you might simply go along with what everyone else desires. However, if you are merely going with the flow, you are not communicating your emotions. Instead, the feelings fester and multiply over weeks, months, and years, transforming into resentment and causing the friendship to steadily deteriorate.

Consider the most recent time someone or several close friends or family members attempted to convince you to do something uncomfortable. What did you do? How did it make you feel? What was the effect on the relationship?

If you've ever felt the pressure of social pressure, you may question how you allowed it to occur. "Am I just not strong enough to say no?" That is not the case. Willpower alone is inadequate. There are numerous reasons why we permit social influences to influence our thoughts, actions, and, ultimately, our interpersonal communication. We conform to the norms of a group in order to acquire acceptance. Because we desire membership in this friend or family group, we readily embrace their rules. Another reason entails the notion of "groupthink." When this occurs, we tend to share the same beliefs as the group and reject criticism from those who disagree with or query the group's behavior. We no longer think independently and instead defer to the group for decisions.

In both cases, social influence is evident. Therefore, the query should not be "How does this happen?" Instead, inquire, "How can I assess how social influence influences my opinions and behaviors? "Are my views truly my own?" Be honest with yourself (which we've learned can be difficult) about how these factors have affected your capacity to communicate in personal relationships.

You should be able to distinguish between your own and social beliefs.

Consider the following concerns regarding social influence.

Which social groups am I a member?

How have my beliefs and behaviors been influenced by these social groups?

How have I communicated my beliefs to these groups as a member?

Reflecting on one's own social beliefs provides valuable insight into the social groups to which one belongs and how these groups influence one's beliefs and behaviors. To prevent social groups from hindering your communication, you must first comprehend what they are. Then you must choose to think independently. This is not to suggest that you disconnect from all social networks; that would be absurd. However, you must be cautious not to lose control of your own decisions and thoughts to those around you. When you are unable to articulate your own thoughts and ideas, you impede communication.

Chapter 9: The Art of Relationship Communication

Connestion: We all srave it. We seek connection through family and acquaintances, but ntmate relationships are frequently where we seek it most. When we fail to do so, we feel alone and misunderstood. We allow these negative emotions to lead to arguments, or worse, we inhibit communication altogether.

Communication is essential to maintaining a strong, healthy relationship. And it isn't about making small talk. Asking your partner how their date went is a pleasant gesture, but if you desire an extraordinary relationship, you must dig deeper. Learning how to communicate in a relationship is about meeting the needs of your companion. To improve communication in your relationship, you must first learn how to listen.

Why Is Communication Important In Relationships?

Communication in relationships is essential for a strong, healthy partnership. Your partner is the person with whom you spend the most time, which increases the risk of miscommunication and misunderstanding. You will be rewarded, however, once you have mastered relationship communication.

_ ENHANCED TRUST

Real communication in a relationship means that you can discuss anything with your partner, including pleasure and sadness, good times and bad. You are willing to be vulnerable with them because you know they will always support and love you. Absolute humiliation and vulnerability is one of the Five Disciplines of Love because it leads to complete trust in your partner.

_ MORE EFFECTIVE CONFLICT RELATIONS

We all know couples who appear to fight constantly and those who appear to never fight. While all relationships experience ur and down, both frequent fghtng and no fghtng at all indicate a lack of communication. The keu is not to disagree with your partner ever. It is to improve your conflict resolution skills by utilizing the eight guidelines listed above so that when disagreements arise, you are able to turn them into something that strengthens your relationship rather than tearing it apart.

_ INCREASED INTIMACY

Discovering how to improve communication in relationships is excellent for your emotional intimacy, or your ability to listen, comprehend, and have compassion for your partner. Developing your communication skills will demonstrate that you respect and value your partner's feelings and opinions. When people feel honored and embraced in this manner, emotional and physical intimacy frequently follow.

4.3 Employ Proper Body Language

Consider the value of nonverbal cues in communication. Consider a group of chimpanzees in a forest as an example. Even though they cannot speak, they communicate primarily through nonverbal cues and body language.

Humans use gesture language and verbal language to communicate, like animals. Consequently, your body posture communicates more than you realize regarding your confidence and commitment in the workplace. The significance of body language stems from its effect on your existence. Positive body language conveys sociability, alertness, and receptivity to new ideas and suggestions.

Frequently, body language is used unconsciously in communication. For instance, if a person yawns or rubs their palm on the table, they will be uninterested and anxious even if the person discusses the established objectives. Conversely, improving your posture gives the impression that you are intrigued and focused. Modify any negative nonverbal cues to improve your self-esteem and confidence. Once you observe others responding positively to you as a friend, employee, or leader, your level of motivation will increase.

In public speaking, the importance of body language is readily apparent. Since all eyes are on them, the individual is under pressure to monitor how much they are speaking and how they should express themselves.

The greeting is an important nonverbal business transaction. Politicians and business leaders seal agreements with handshakes. A firm handshake communicates assurance, whereas a feeble handshake indicates apathy.

Remember to smile and sustain eye contact during handshakes. This demonstrates your courage and confidence. If you have a habit of clenching your fists or wiping your eyes, be conscious of it and replace it with a rhythmic body movement.

Texting and Internet courtship

When communicating via text, there are no facial expressions or body language cues to indicate what the other person is thinking or feeling. When two people have not yet met in person, there is no knowledge to enlighten assumptions; therefore, when reading texts, we rely on our imagination. Therefore, it is essential to pay attention to the language and tone of your messages. Be extremely aware of the possibility of miscommunication, and grant the other person the benefit of the doubt.

Texting can help you better understand someone's demeanor and communication style. It can also be a fun way to flirt, develop rapport, and maintain the flow of conversation. Using optimistic language will aid in establishing a strong connection with your potential partner. If you need assistance starting a conversation, try asking your date open-ended queries that will encourage them to share more about themselves.

Although face-to-face communication is preferable, it is not always feasible. This method of communication is based on the notion that words can evoke strong emotional responses in others. In other words, by meticulously choosing our words, we can affect how others perceive us.

Use these three techniques to enhance the persuasiveness of your writing:

1. Send positive messages: Be careful to send upbeat and optimistic messages. Negativity will only serve to repel the other person. If you have a sardonic sense of humor, reserve it for in-person interactions. Text does not translate

sarcasm well, particularly if you do not know each other.

Choose your words with care, and use language that is forceful and emotive. Words are extremely potent, so use them judiciously! Consider carefully before texting something that could have multiple meanings; use words that are crystal clear.

3. Employ active voice: Avoid passive language and phrases such as "I believe" and "perhaps we could." Use active phrases such as "I'd love to see that exhibit, would you like to join?" or "Why don't we try the new restaurant?" This manner of speech conveys interest and determination.

Text Messaging and Romantic Partnerships

Modern couples are nearly as likely to communicate through a screen as they are face-to-face. Texting can be a practical method of communication, but it can also present new challenges.

Couples may argue via text message or use text to resume an already tense conversation that began in person. Given how readily texts can be misunderstood, they have the potential to spark explosive misunderstandings. Texting may also hinder the ability of couples to communicate effectively. It can be simple for messages to get lost in translation when attempting to communicate complex emotions or topics via text. Texting to continue an argument that began in person is a recipe for disaster and should be avoided.

Numerous emotional aspects of conflict resolution cannot be conveyed via text message. If you are prone to exchanging impassioned texts with anyone in your life, consider the number of arguments you've settled via text. Any? Or, does messaging simply prolong the conversation until an impasse is reached and the issue is resolved in a subsequent conversation?

Despite the difficulties that messaging can pose for romantic relationships, there are also some positive aspects. Texting is an excellent method for maintaining contact with your companion throughout the day. It is also a useful method of communication when you cannot speak on the phone or meet in person. In addition, messaging can foster intimacy and connection in a relationship when used appropriately.

Obviously, there are exceptions to the norm. Some individuals find it more convenient to communicate via text because it allows them to consider their words without being interrupted. This can facilitate more meaningful and reflective conversations. Texting can be positive or negative for romantic relationships, depending on how it is utilized. Texting can be a wonderful tool for fostering intimacy and connection if used thoughtfully and with consideration for your partner's needs.

Chapter 10: The some essential methods to express affection are affirming words, deeds of service

It is essential to understand your own way of expressing affection and that of your partner. As individuals, we have various primary avenues for affection. The primary channels of affection reveal the actuality of our emotions.

Some relationships fail because the two players don't comprehend their partner's main avenues for affection. They may be communicating love through their own main avenues for affection rather than their partner's, causing their partner to feel unappreciated, which is undesirable in a relationship.

Expressions of devotion

Positive Affirmations

Few of us genuinely enjoy hearing sweet phrases such as "I love you" and "I adore the dress you wore last night." Not that they didn't already know that their partner adores them, but those words continually renew their affection for their partner. I like that you don't have to actually see your partner in order to express your feelings through uplifting words.

Volunteer Service

Some individuals are not moved by straightforward words; they prefer activities because they recognize that talk is cheap. Those in this category merely require assistance or administrations to be administered to them. For instance, if your partner is a fashion designer, assisting them with ironing their garments or anything else related to their design work will go a long way with them.

Gifts

Almost everyone values this, so if you know that your partner's primary expression of devotion is through gifts, pick up a bouquet of chocolates and roses the next time you're out and give them to them; this will make them feel cherished.

cherished leisure

Not everyone has sufficient time outside of their busy schedules to spend with their partner, but the time you do spend with them is extremely important to them. It isn't necessary to see each other in person throughout everything involving extra effort, video calls, talking, and audio cause can go quite far.

actual contact

If you believe that your partner is generally at ease when caressed, then that may be their way of expressing affection; some may prefer kisses or embraces, while others may simply want to feel your body around them.

It is essential to identify and comprehend your partner's primary mode of devotion.

There is no perfect relationship, but with the right partner, you can have the practically perfect relationship you crave.

Chapter 11: How To Commence And Continue A Conversation

It could be intimidating to initiate communication with a stranger. Here are some tips on how to carry on a conversation like a pro in order to establish those crucial relationships.

What Constitutes a Good Discussion?

Numerous factors contribute to an engaging discussion. Listed below are some factors that can prevent awkward silences.

1. attentive hearing

Active listening emphasizes paying close attention to what is being said when another person is speaking. Sometimes people listen in order to respond to what their conversation partner is saying, as opposed to hearing what their conversation companion is saying.

If you employ this essential strategy, your discussion companion will recognize that you are attentive. Additionally, you will likely recall more of the conversation subsequently. By speaking less and listening more, repeating what you have just heard to the speaker, and engaging in active listening, you may be able to enhance your listening skills.

2. Posing and responding to queries

Another way to demonstrate that you are a good listener is to ask inquiries.

You can extend the conversation by asking questions about what the other individual said. Alternatively, you may inquire about anything you were unsure of or wish to learn more about.

Again, this demonstrates to the other individual your genuine interest in what they have to say.

3. discovering similar interests and traits

Listen attentively throughout conversations to identify shared experiences. You can keep the conversation flowing naturally by bringing up shared interests, which will provide you with topics to discuss.

Finding common ground will help you initiate a fruitful conversation. This is essential for maintaining the rhythm of the conversation.

Having a purpose for the conversation

Before beginning a conversation, it's typically a good idea to have a plan, whether you've run into a friend at the supermarket or at a networking event.

If you have a clear objective, the conversation will have direction and won't feel uneasy or awkward.

If you observe that the conversation is lagging, you may use its purpose to introduce a new topic of discussion.

Chapter 12: How to effectively communicate, actively listen, and interpret body language

Here are some suggestions for enhancing your communication abilities. You can become a better observer, speaker, and communicator by following these tips.

Once upon a time, there was a youthful CEO who was terrible at listening, speaking, and communicating. He was perpetually misunderstood and never seemed to communicate effectively.

One day, he decided to attempt to improve his situation, so he enrolled in a communication seminar. The seminar spanned an entire weekend, and he was determined to learn and take advantage of the opportunity.

He was astounded by how much he had learned during the seminar. He learned the significance of active listening, how to effectively convey himself, how to interpret body language, and how to tell stories, among other things.

He promptly applied what he had learned because he was so enthusiastic about it. The more he paid attention to what others were saying, the better he was able to comprehend them. In addition, he became more confident and articulate when expressing his views.

As a result of the seminar and the knowledge he acquired, he felt so empowered. He was now confident in his abilities and able to effectively communicate with those around him.

You are about to receive the same seminar as a chapter.

How to Locate the Finest Employees

How do you determine who would be a decent addition to your team when you receive fifty or more resumes from job-seekers? Consider their educational background, such as the universities they attended. Or how many years of work experience they have? Many leaders have kicked themselves after realizing that just because someone has a degree in the field or more than five years of experience in the field does not mean they know how to perform their task. It relates back to our discussion of cognitive fallacies, specifically the halo effect.

When searching for the best employees, the trick is to spend less time perusing their impressive titles and more time searching for indicators of good character. You can mimic a variety of things, but character is extremely difficult to imitate. The character of a job candidate defines who they are, how they view the world, and what they value. By practicing discriminate listening and observing nonverbal signals, you can learn a great deal about the character of a job applicant.

I will never forget when I was recruiting a marketing manager many years ago. Candidates were required to record a three-minute video introducing themselves as part of the screening procedure. In the midst of their presentation, a young person took a massive yawn and continued as if nothing had happened.

In any other setting, it would have been amusing and I wouldn't give it much thought. However, because this recording was part of their interview, it taught me a great deal about their personality. I assumed they were too indolent to re-record and lacked the self-awareness to comprehend how unprofessional it was. Regardless, I did not want that type of employee on my team, particularly at a managerial level!

In his book The Ideal Team Player, Patrick Lencioni identifies three qualities that employees must possess in order to be effective team players: humility, desire, and intelligence (Lencioni, 2016). He explains that these traits foster accountability, constructive conflict resolution, dedication, and improved work performance. Below is a summary of each characteristic:

Humility

The definition of humility is having a modest opinion of oneself. This typically entails putting the requirements of the company or team ahead of your own in the workplace. When there is work to be done, you offer your assistance to the best of your ability without pursuing credit. A humble employee prioritizes team goals and looks for ways to make the team appear good.

Hunger

Demonstrating hunger requires a commitment to learn and develop. You are eager to participate in endeavors that challenge your intellect, necessitate extensive investigation, or involve solving problems. An employee who demonstrates appetite is self-motivated and dedicated to serving others. They are motivated by their long-term objectives and the desire to improve themselves.

Intelligence

When you consider intellect in the workplace, you should not think of someone who is book smart. Consider instead a person who aspires for excellence in all endeavors and possesses exceptional emotional intelligence and interpersonal skills. They are intelligent because they intuitively know what actions and behaviors are appropriate in every circumstance. They are excellent listeners, assertive communicators, and have a knack for bringing team members together (they are typically well-known and likable).

Please note that an applicant's character alone is sufficient to gain employment. In addition to character, you must ensure that the candidate is qualified and a good cultural fit. By cultural fit, I mean that when speaking with a candidate, you feel an immediate rapport and get the impression that they would get along well with other team members. Since the advent of the hybrid work schedule, chemistry may no longer be a priority for many organizations, but there will be times when collaboration is required and employees must work productively together.

All of this sifting and filtering will ultimately lead to the interview phase. Depending on how the recruitment procedure is structured, there will not be many candidates to interview. This is excellent news, as it gives you a bit more time to study each candidate, ask insightful questions, and gauge that all-important chemistry!

If you want to maximize the effectiveness of your interviews, you should avoid the standard question-and-answer format. Currently, candidates are aware of the types of questions asked by recruiters, and they typically obtain a cheat sheet and practice their answers the night before an interview. You don't strike me as the type of leader who hires employees who cut corners, so look for impromptu methods to facilitate the interview. Here are some helpful suggestions:

Acting out a role. Create common workplace scenarios and ask the candidate to demonstrate how they would respond to or resolve the presented challenges if employed. For instance, a candidate being interviewed for a customer service position may be asked to handle an irate caller.

Introduce a problem that they must solve. Assess the candidate's problem-solving skills by presenting them with a typical obstacle they may confront in their new position. Consider various factors, such as how they respond to pressure, implement their skills, think creatively, and employ tried-and-true techniques.

Public Presentations: Inform the interviewee a few days or weeks before the scheduled interview that they will need to have a presentation prepared. If you want the presentation to contain specific elements, provide explicit instructions (and perhaps some examples). While it is recommended to have real-time presentations so that you can evaluate nonverbal cues and get a feel for the person, you can also request that they record their presentations and transmit them to you by a certain date.

● Engage in a coffee rendezvous. Since you are not in an office environment, taking the interviewee out for coffee can help to put them at ease. Nonetheless, you are able to observe how they interact with waiters, express their thoughts, and manage casual small talk. This is probably the best method to determine whether you have chemistry with the candidate and whether you can work with them on a daily basis.

Introduce them to an existing team member. It can be advantageous to introduce a candidate to someone with whom they will interact closely. It will not only prevent cognitive bias, but also assist you in determining whether the candidate is a good cultural fit. If the current employee raises red flags, you may reconsider whether they are the best candidate for the position.

Creatively designed interviews can elicit more information from candidates. Do not misunderstand; the purpose is not to intimidate the candidate or place them on the spot. The objective is to encourage the candidate to be authentic and not rely on a script to make the best impression. In addition to evaluating the corporation during the interview, candidates also evaluate the organization. Yes, they are observing how hard you work to discover qualified candidates. During the interview process, you want to emphasize your company's mission and core values in order to inspire candidates about working for you.

Important to effective communication is attentive attention. It involves actively hearing to and comprehending the viewpoints of others, as opposed to merely waiting your turn to speak.

Active listening necessitates effort and vigilance, but it can greatly improve communication and strengthen relationships.

In this chapter, we will discuss the advantages of active listening and how to implement it in our everyday interactions.

Body:

Advantages of vigilant listening:

The benefits of active listening extend to both the observer and the speaker.

Active listening facilitates the development of trust, comprehension, and rapport between the receiver and the speaker. It also enables the listener to gather additional information and gain a better understanding of the speaker's viewpoint.

Active listening can validate the speaker's thoughts and emotions, allowing them to feel heard and understood. It can also assist the speaker in clarifying their thoughts and gaining a better understanding of their own emotions and requirements.

Active listening can enhance communication and strengthen relationships in general.

Strategies for active listening practice:

There are a number of techniques you can use to practice active listening:

Avoid distractions, such as checking your phone or multitasking, and focus on the speaker.

Use nonverbal cues, such as sustaining eye contact and nodding, to demonstrate that you are attentive and listening to the speaker.

Do not interrupt or speak over the speaker. Wait for them to complete their thought before responding.

Use clarifying queries to demonstrate interest and an effort to comprehend. For instance, "Could you tell me more about that?" or "Could you give me an example of what you mean?"

Restate what you have heard to demonstrate comprehension. For instance: "What I heard you say was..."

Conclusion:

Active listening is an essential component of effective communication that can significantly enhance relationships and comprehension.

By paying close attention, asking clarifying questions, and engaging in self-reflection, we can practice active listening and enhance our communication abilities.

Two or three suggestions for removing suspicion:

1) have reservations about reusing data. Consider it while contemplating other factors, and do not become involved unless you have proof. It is easy to latch onto something we "need" to hear, and this is precisely the danger.

2) Be informed while adopting. In the event that you had no notion or did not hear it yourself, you are accepting. This includes some degree of anticipation. If you see something, it may not tell the whole story (such as what Jill's companion observed). Avoid using a scene as inspiration for your own writing.

 Moreover, assumptions about relationships can be especially

destructive, wreaking havoc in your work, family, and public activities. [Are you unsure of what a secure relationship is? Peruse our Guide to Excellent Relationships. How do suspicions appear? He did not call me this evening, indicating that he is not interested. Never assume you know how another person thinks and feels, because you see things through the lens of your unique perspective and value system, which are rarely identical to the next person's. Observable facts about a situation or a person's actions can be known, but a person's feelings and thoughts are only accessible if you ask them. Moreover, they should have enough faith in you to tell you the truth. Not sure if you're making a guess or not? Ask yourself the subsequent: What evidence do I need to demonstrate the validity of this belief? What evidence do I need to demonstrate that this belief is false? Is it my own perception, or did someone else inform me of this and I assumed it to be true? Likewise, consider what others say in your connections. Do you frequently hear, "Stop telling me what you're thinking"? Have people ever told you, "You are constantly speaking for me?" Or, conversely, do companions and partners say things like, "You generally assume you know how I feel when you don't?" Then, examine expressions that demonstrate assumptions, such as "I'm certain that...", "I can tell that...", "I simply have a hunch that...", and "obviously, he/she..." Assumptions result in 'close down'. As a result of our own presumptions, we cease being open and responsive to the next individual, cease endeavoring to interact, cease exerting effort, and may even end a relationship. Suppositions make consistent duress and struggle . If we assume we know what another person is thinking or why they did what they did, they may feel judged, trapped, or as if they are rarely given opportunities. If you consistently harbor suspicions about others, you may appear to be extremely cautious. Even without trying, you might be perceived as severe. In addition, assumptions can leave you feeling discreetly very despondent. They construct a barrier around you, leaving others on the outside. How could I consistently speculate? It is not surprising due to the need to exert control over others and circumstances. If not knowing how others think and feel makes you feel vulnerable, suspicions help you regain a sense of control over everything. Assumptions can also serve as a method for avoiding localized torment. By constantly assuming we comprehend what others think and feel, we avoid the risk of being defenseless. We reject input that could be harmful, but in doing so, we also tragically miss out on learning the positive things others may wish to teach us, such as authentic affection and love. Consequently, individuals with a fear of proximity frequently engage in the practice of speculation. However, if you believe you can't stop driving others away and your tendency to make outlandish assumptions, you should seek professional help. So aside. Insofar as this specific trade is concerned, it is a presumption to inquire whether it is one of several items. You are assuming it is either/or and attempting to control the outcome by presenting two options, despite the fact that you are not in the other person's mind and have no idea about the many possible reasons.